I0790812

MINDFUL MASTURBATION FOR MEN!

Goddess Leianna

Dedication

To all my wonderful clients
throughout the years who have supported and
followed me; and, to those to come.
Thank you for honoring, appreciating, and
worshipping the Divine Feminine.

This book is for you!

Contents

1. Set the Stage

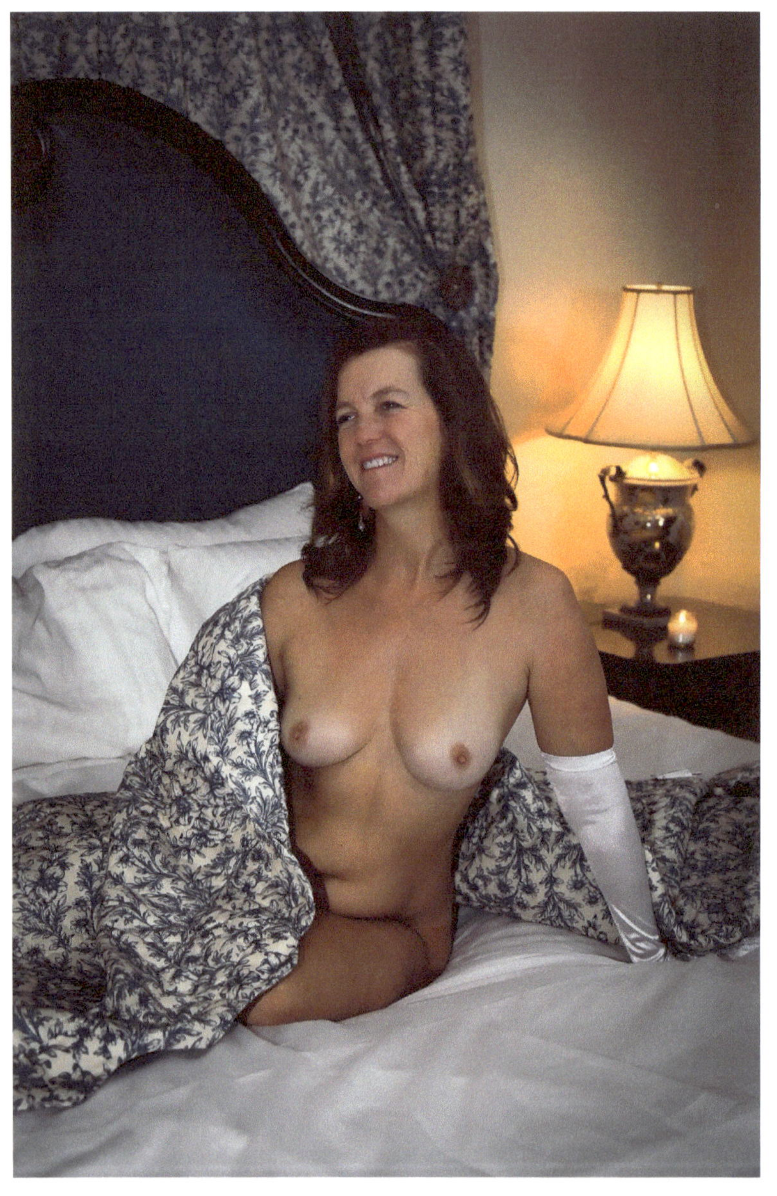

Gentlemen!
Good vibes happen in sexy space!
Make sure yours is ready.
Tidy your space;
light the candles;
clear the air by burning incense or sage;
and intend for an incredible
erotic journey.

2. Undress

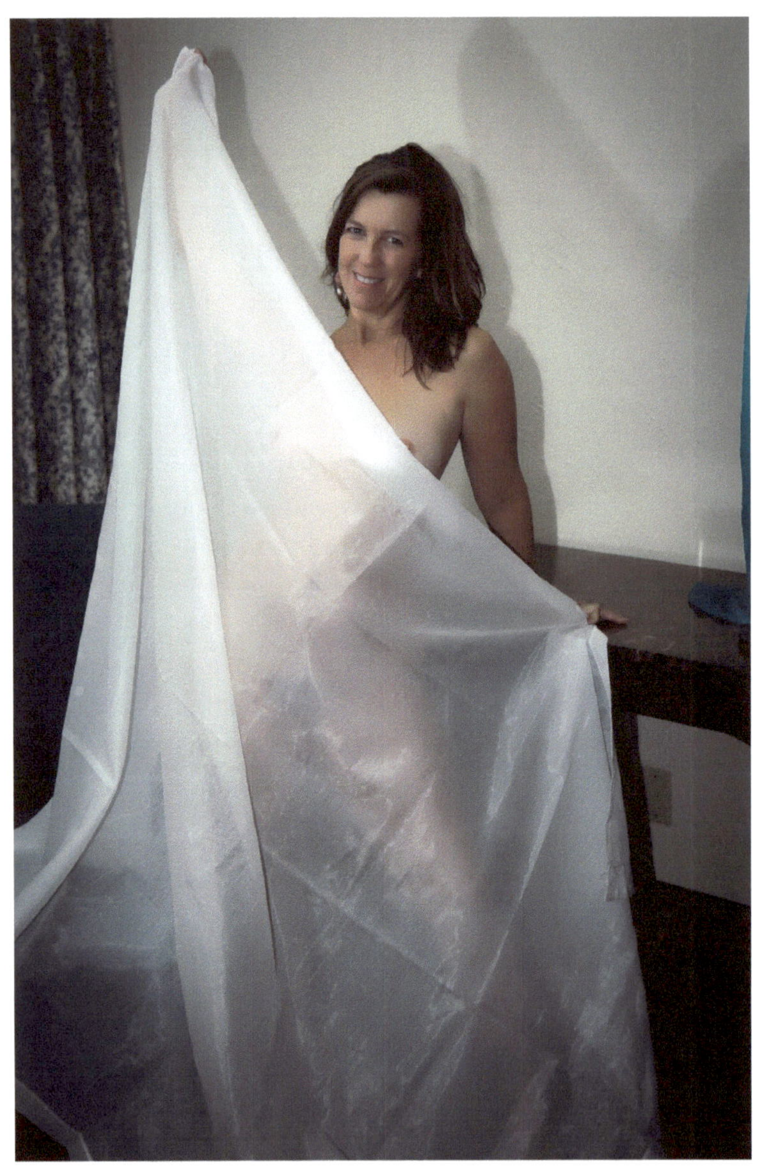

Stand in your sacred space and
slowly begin to feel your clothing.
Feel the textures, the linen,
and, loosen that tie around your neck.
Begin to peel the layers of the day off your body.
Remove that shirt.
Feel the air as it touches your naked skin,
perking up your nipples.
Feel the coolness on your neck.
Now, unbuckle those pants, take notice of your handsome
Cock. It's yours.
Slide those britches down and drop them,
feel your masculine exposed and available.
Dream about those sexy women who want to reach out and
touch that beautiful organ.

3. Ground Yourself

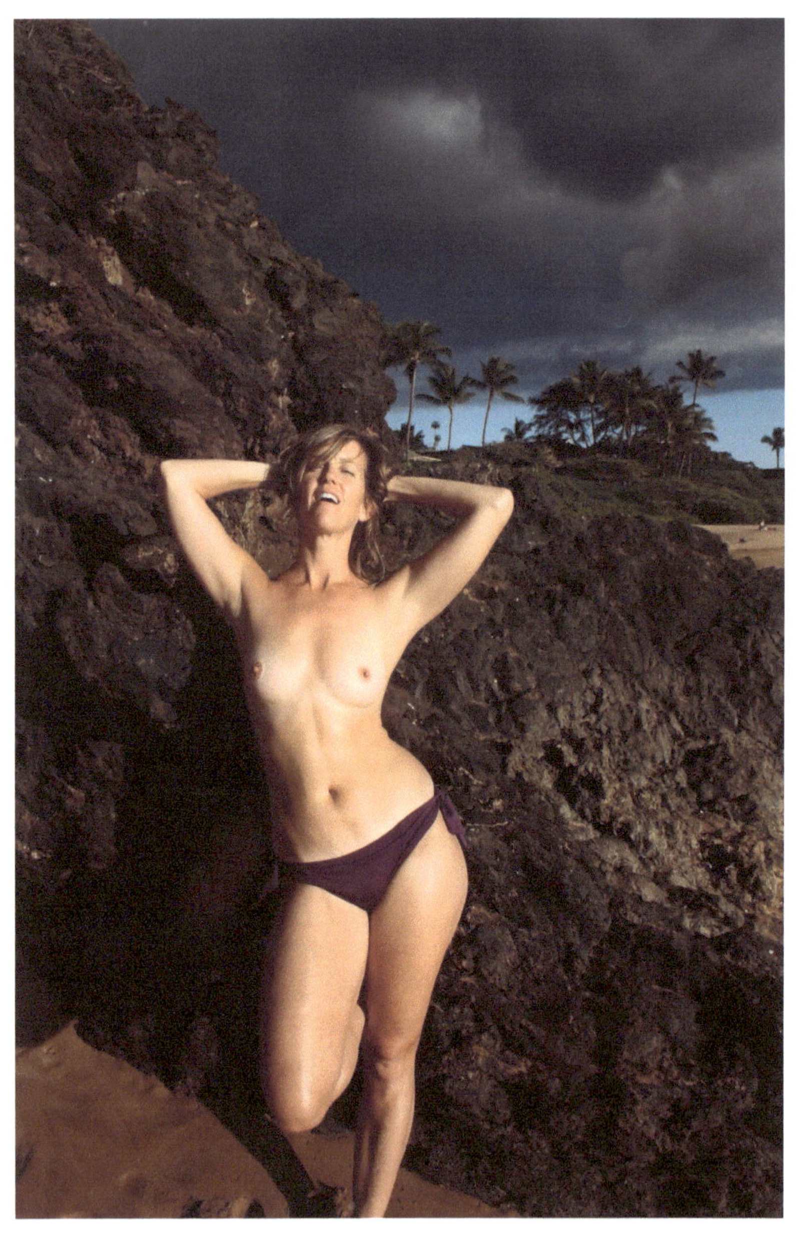

Feel where you are in the moment.

Take notice of your surroundings.

Smell the air and the scent of you.

Sense that throbbing in your organ and the growl in your stomach hungry for something tantalizing and thrilling.

Imagine.

This will be best masturbation ever!

You are the Master!

You make it happen!

4. *Meditate*

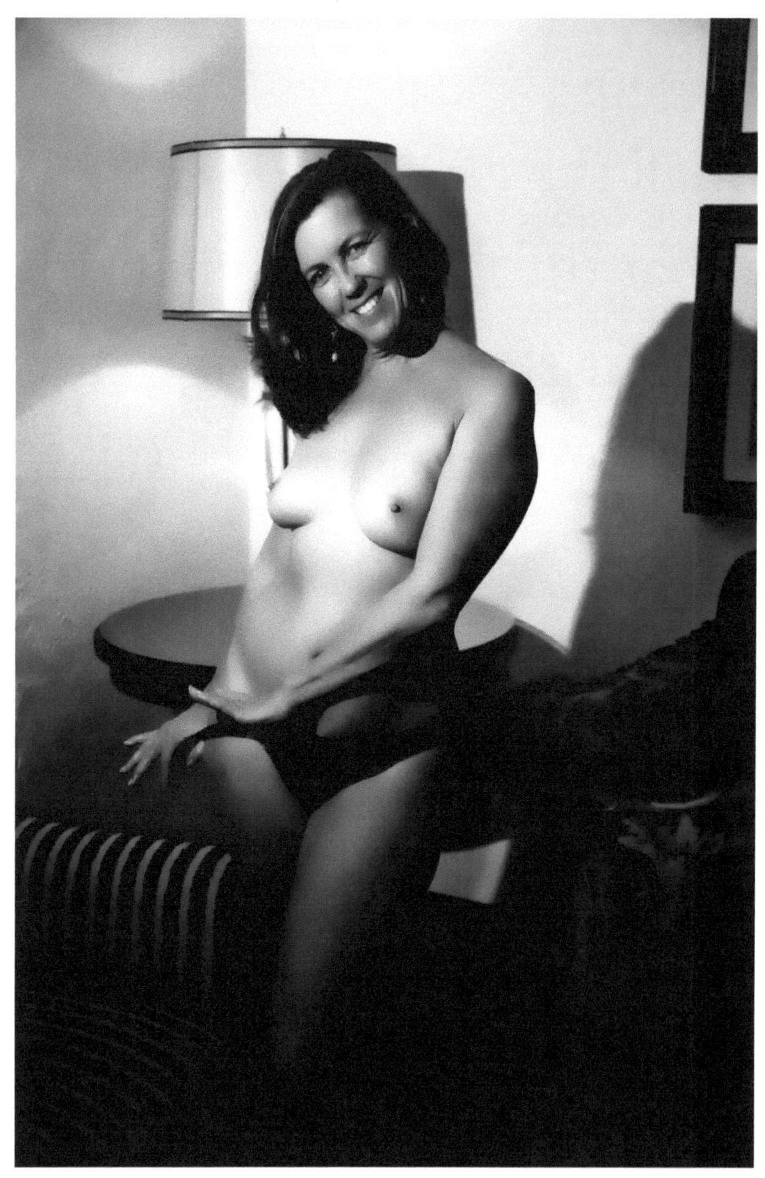

Listen to your breath; clear your head.

Ask for the daily chores and the
unfinished "to do" list to leave you.

Be free of worries.

Let go.

Sit in a comfortable position.

Slowly inhale; breathe in that Spirit;
notice your essence as the Man you are!

Hold still; quiet the mind; breathe slowly.

Empty out the contents of your briefcase,
work pad, or notebook.

Say goodbye to your clients, your customers, and
your boss!

5. Breathe

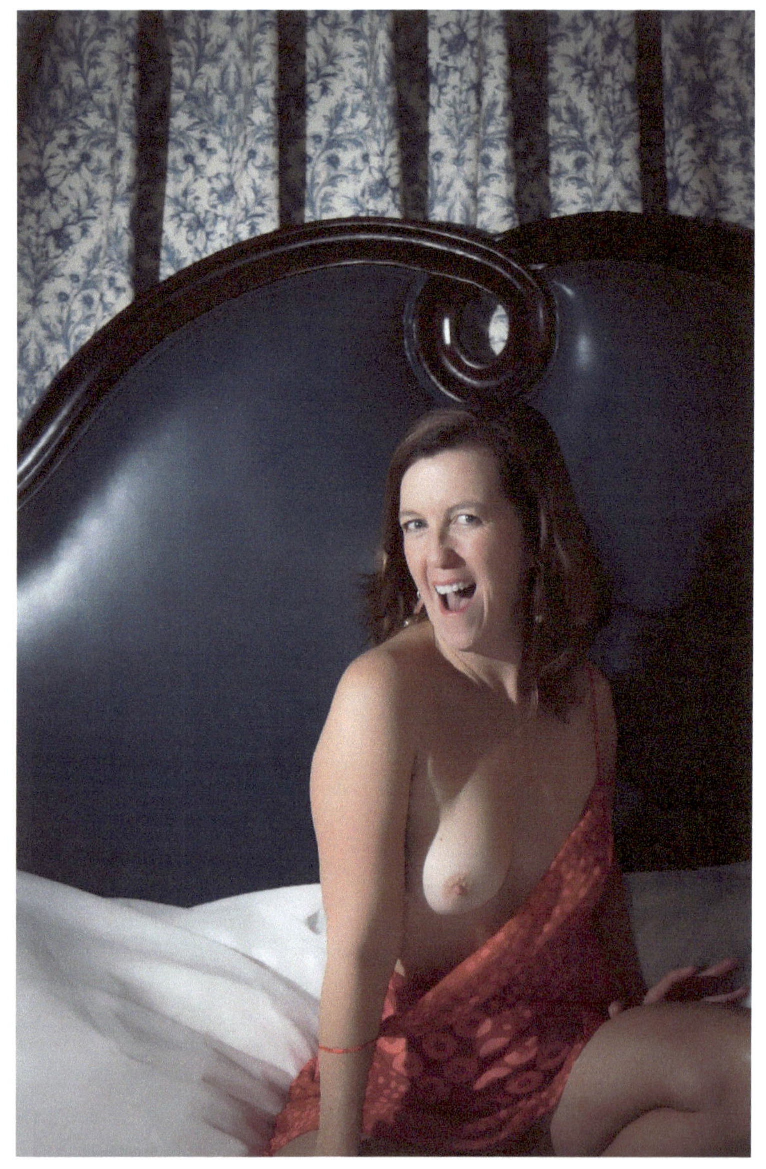

Allow your breath to enter and fill your belly.

Fill you with you.

Inhale deeply through the nose.

Exhale now with a full charged breath as

in a "HA!"

Give it all you've got.

Inhale the fullness of your masculine.

Exhale the charge in your belly.

Exhale the stress of the day.

Relax.

6. Feel

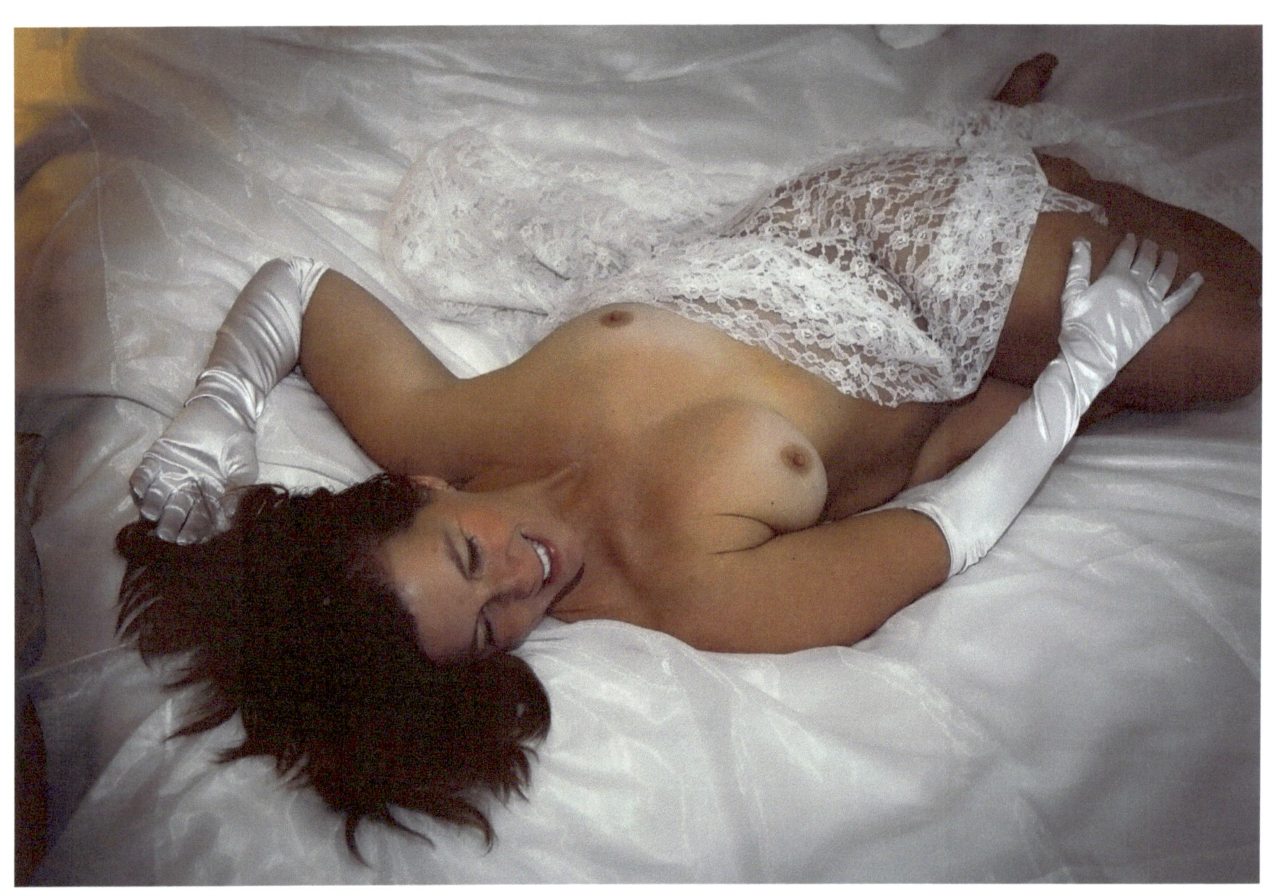

Feel your chest. Take notice of the hair or the
waxed surface.
Slowly make contact with your awakened hands.
Feel your arms.
Run your hand up and over to the other arm.
Appreciate your facial hair. The texture.
Is it smooth, silky, or rough like you?
Touch that sexy hair of yours.
Feel your legs, your inner thighs, your buttocks.
Keep your hands moving everywhere…
…except your Cock.
Leave it alone.
Be Patient.

7. Stroke

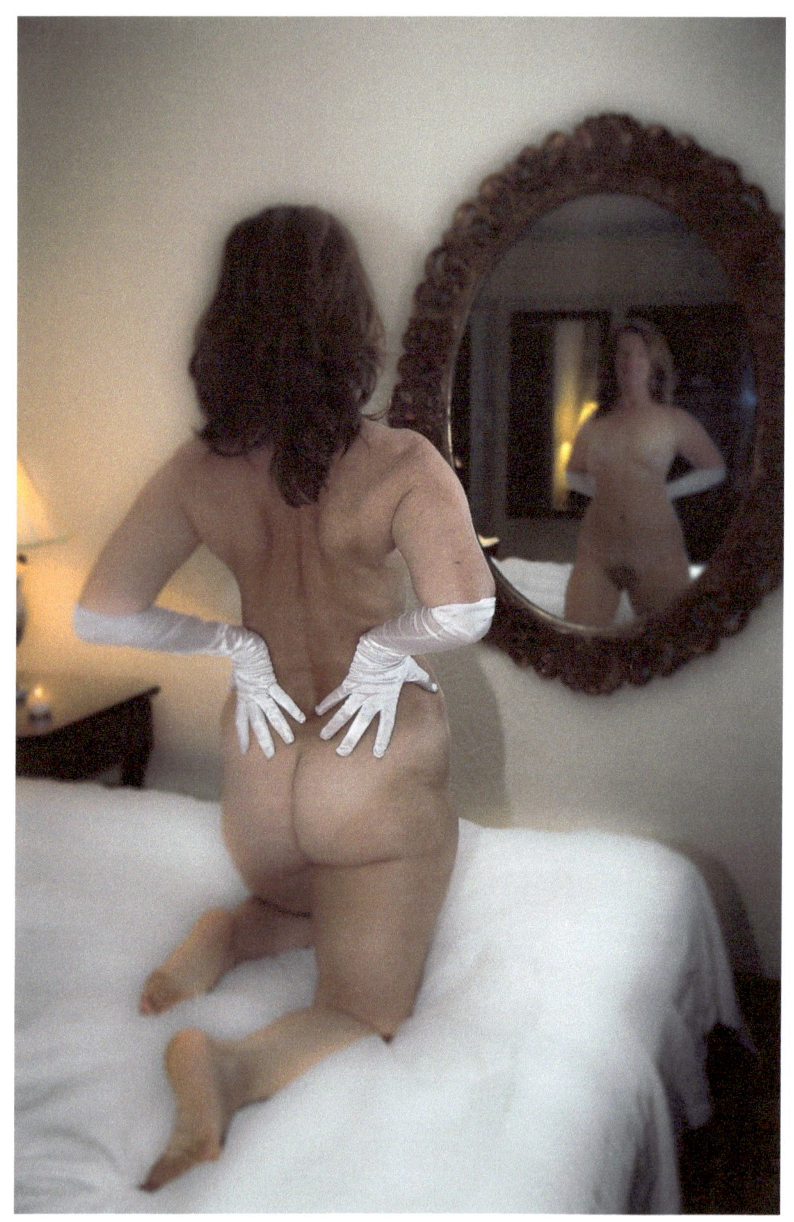

Now. Gently move your hands to your Cock.
Touch the head, the front, the back.
Notice how hard you are.
Slowly grip it with your whole being with
all of your attention.
Its been a long day…hold it tight.
Take your hands and find your balls, gently grab
them bit by bit, pulling the skin away from the
middle, stretching it.
Rub it, tug it, gently caress.
Breathe in the sensations.
Exhale the charge.

8. Feel again

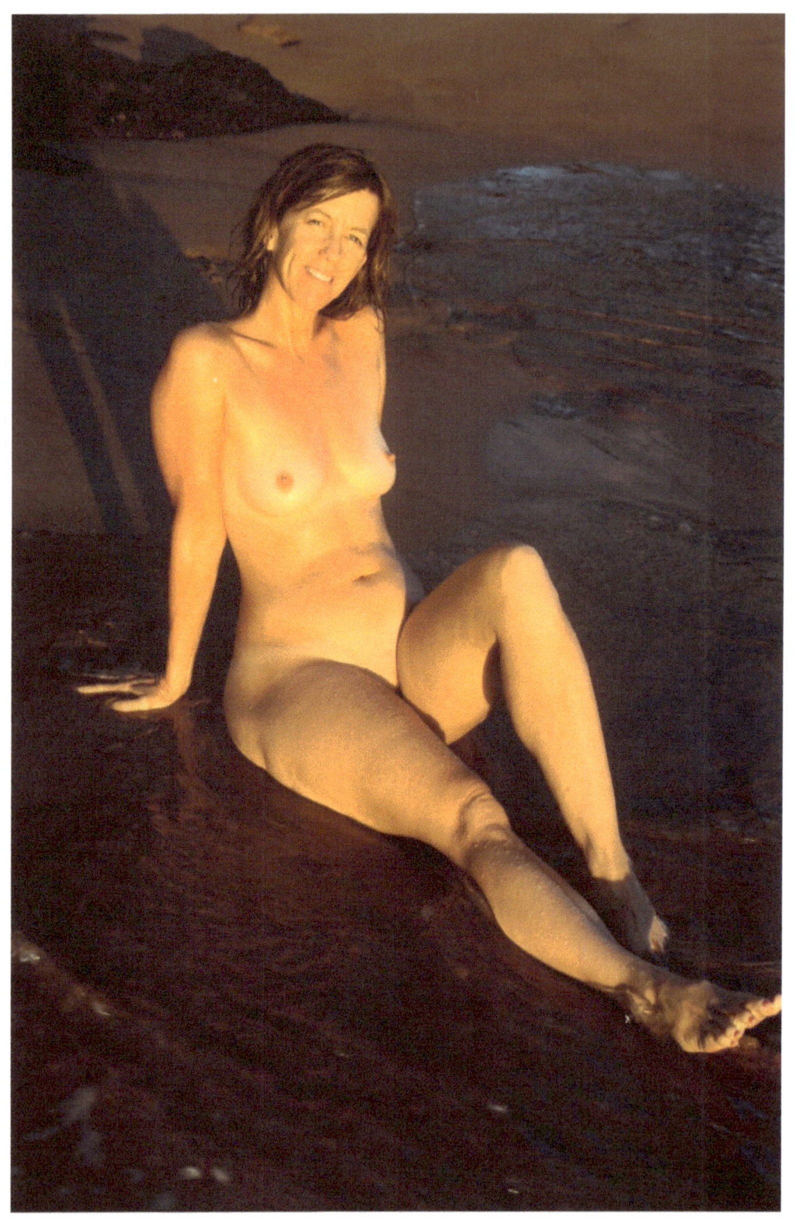

Notice your mouth…feel the watering sensation,
open your mouth…
let the sound of pleasure be expelled.
Really…let it Go!
Feel the vibration in your belly. Can it vibrate even
more as you express your pleasure even louder?
Feel the ripples on your skin;
the hair gently vibrating.
Inhale and move your erotic energy up through
your heart and throat.
Imagine it moving out of the top of the head.
Create a circle of yummy energy
moving around you and through you.
You've got this!

9. Build the Energy

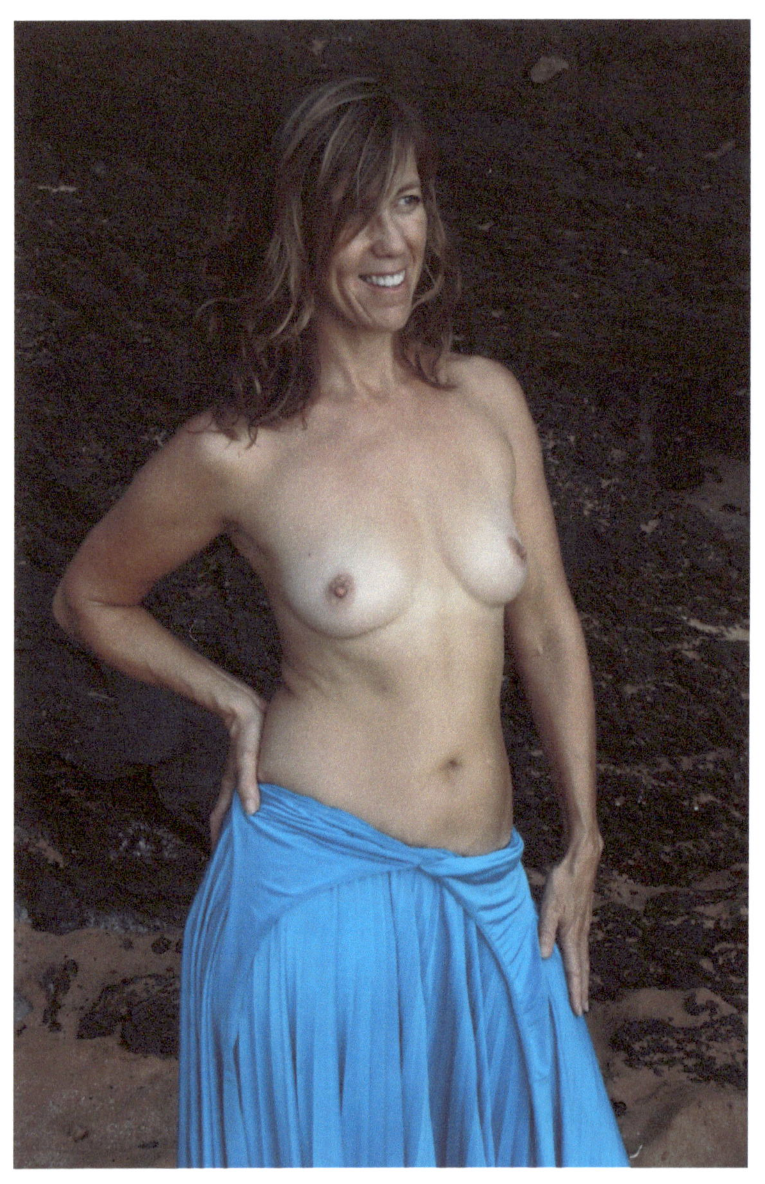

Quicken your breath, your stroke.

Inhale really deep, now exhale again.

Keep the breath moving with the
rhythm of your stroke.

Stay focused on what you are feeling.

Intending what you want.

To expand everywhere!

Do not wander anywhere.

Look at me.

Stay with me.

Stroke Baby.

Build the energy…now let it go… build again….let
it go…build and build…build
AHHHHHH!

10. Release

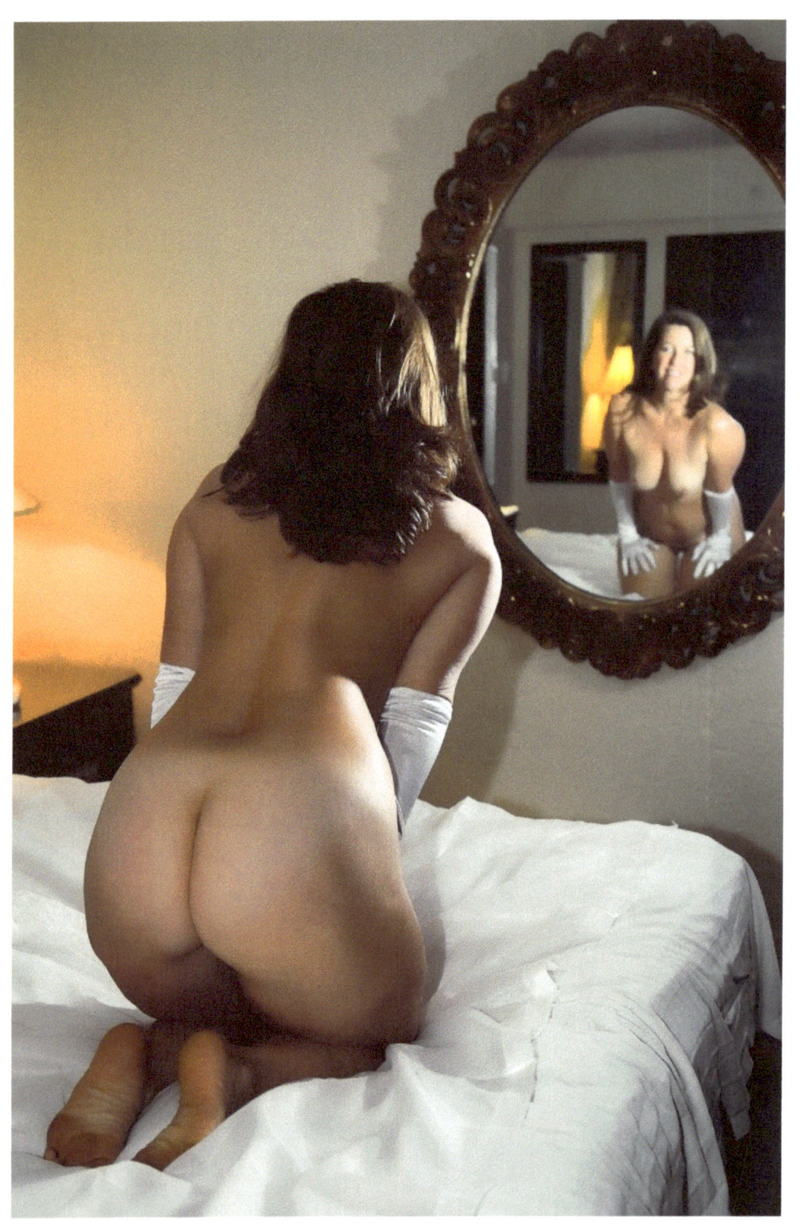

Here it is handsome.

A nice big Orgasm, just for you!

Allow the pulsations of waves to wash over
and engulf you.

Breathing always…moving your energy,
take it right to the very last minute.

Remain as One with your Orgasm.

You've earned it!

Stay with it.

Breathe into it.

Vibrate.

BE!

Now Rest.

About Your Goddess

Goddess Leianna is a mature, lovely, intelligent Goddess
who has made her way in life pursuing her dreams and
touching whom she pleases.
She is sexy, savvy and sassy, as well as,
very sacred and spiritual.
Her mission with this book,
is to take you on your own personal sacred journey,
allowing you to come home to yourself again and again,
finding inner peace through a mindful masturbation.

Namaste!